The Window Of My Soul

The Window Of My Soul

ALISON MURPHY

Dedication

To my friends and family and the medical team who have supported me so well throughout my illness.

THE WINDOW OF MY SOUL
Copyright © 2022 by Alison Murphy

ISBN 978-1-915223-17-3

Published by

Maurice Wylie Media
Inspirational Christian Publisher

For more information visit:
www.MauriceWylieMedia.com

Contents

Introduction

As I sit here finishing off my first book, I cannot believe that I have reached the milestone of 60 years old.

I was raised in Belfast but have lived for the last 20 years in Comber which have been my happiest.

After a very traumatic period, at the age of 27, I was diagnosed with schizophrenia and then later at the age of 57, I was diagnosed with cancer.

I have had a difficult life, however with an amazing and supportive husband, there were many happy memories.

I am a very deep, sensitive person and I have written eleven stories and twelve poems in a very truthful and personal way about my life and my cancer journey, and my unshakeable Christian faith.

My hope is that whoever reads my accounts of life's difficulties will be taken down a path which will hopefully lead you to a personal relationship with The Lord Jesus Christ.

I also hope you will find hope and comfort knowing that you are not alone. It is meant especially for the lonely, the mentally ill, people with and caring for cancer, and for people who are searching for the truth about a living and wonderful Heavenly father.

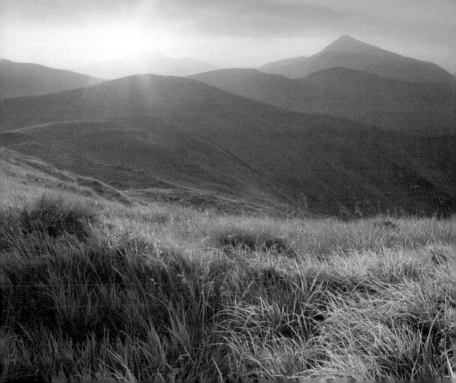

SECTION ONE

Stories

1

The Butterfly

'I'm not sure I want to get this tattoo,' I said to Lorraine.

'Come on Ali, the girl has been waiting half an hour, go ahead … oh, by the way, the tattoo is four inches long.' *Four inches,* I thought, boy, I knew I would really regret this, but as usual I couldn't say no — not to anyone.

Just the same as a few other things in my life, the tattoo was something I regretted at the time, but I have come to see a deeper meaning, which I believe was planned.

Six months later, I was in my doctor's surgery, and he was staring at the tattoo, that strangely I had come to love. He sat back in the chair and spoke. 'Alison, it will have to come off, you are allergic to the ink.'

I was shocked and felt a surge of disappointment. I was looking forward to wearing cropped trousers and showing it off this summer.

The laser treatment finished last year but now, in 2022, the tattoo is red and itchy, but I think with a little TLC, it will be okay.

In May 2019, I had a different problem and the tattoo felt as though it was more than a nuisance — I discovered I had cancer of the mouth.

It's now 2022. I'm not in remission yet, but I'm a fighter of the first degree, and have fought this cancer with every blood vessel in my body. And just as there are still problems with my tattoo, there are also problems with my mouth.

The situation has changed and so have I. My diet is liquid and I no longer speak as I used to, but my core is still there, the part of you that never dies — the spirit that lives on.

And just like a butterfly, I started my life as an egg. And as a caterpillar crawls on its belly, the first half of my life had many difficulties. Life was definitely a struggle. Caterpillars are vulnerable, sensitive little insects — as was I.

Cancer; however, changed me. From being a shy, awkward girl, sadly, I became a shy, awkward woman.

Suddenly, through cancer, there was a transition.

I'm not exactly sure why, but not only was I changing outwardly after losing four stone in weight, but inwardly the beauty of Christ was beginning to appear.

Spiritually, I felt like a new person. I have experienced an amazing transformation. Some people might say I'm vain because I'm so interested in my appearance. I say *I am happy* and beauty lies deep within a person.

I might look and dress younger than my age, but those lines on my face and neck tell a completely different story — a story of hardship, trials, illness and much more.

Hope is something I hold on to. It is the fundamental belief that most people live by. I am nearly sixty years old, but I *hope* I live another ten years, as a butterfly, metaphorically speaking.

And finally life. Well the nurses and doctors have worked tirelessly to give me back my life, and God has seen to it that my life has been preserved, at least for now.

The tattoo is still itchy, but the red, dry skin reminds me of what I have come through and what I have become. The scar is left for all to see.

And just as a butterfly's life is short-lived, who knows, mine could be also. That's a matter for the highest of hands.

2

The Window Of My Soul

My soul is the deepest immortal part of me, the most sensitive part that has battled through a life of adversity. God has taken it and made it strong and resilient.

Here is a little window that will take you down a path that will hopefully lead you to a place of peace which is where I am now.

I think it is normal for me to hold out my hands and look up to the heavens and ask the question, 'Why me?' And for the people who may say, 'Why not me?' When you have had to face the challenges, trials and insults I have, comments like that don't always help.

When I was thirty-four, I fell out with God. I became angry, and in my ignorance and inexperience, I said things I definitely shouldn't have. There is absolutely no point in doing that, it achieves nothing; it damages your relationship with God and leaves you feeling a loneliness that cannot be compared to any other.

As I approach my sixtieth birthday, I can honestly say I have found peace, which I don't think would have happened except through my journey with cancer.

It is of significance that I was diagnosed with schizophrenia at the age of twenty-seven. During my lifetime I have had many bad and some disturbing experiences, but when I see the power of God with my cancer, I can only hold up my hands and praise him for his unshakeable faithfulness to me.

The friends he has brought me, the prayers that have been said, and the prayers that have been answered over and over again.

My soul has learnt that sometimes you have to say goodbye to people and that doesn't necessarily mean they have died.

It is very important to line up your life to the life God has planned for you. No other way will work out for the best.

It's good to be assertive and speak the truth and to always be able to have your say but to accept that other people have a say also.

My soul has been humbled on many occasions and said sorry for wrong doings. A number of people don't accept apologies. That is a matter between them and God and not something I dwell on.

My soul belongs to The Lord, I will never lose sight of that. He holds me steadfast and he loves me and has always protected me.

Through many dangers, toils and snares, I have already come. I sing this hymn and have had first-hand experience of all those things.

God never said we would have a trouble-free life but promised to be with us in it, right in the very heart and depth of what we are going through. Someday, when I meet him, I will sob tears of happiness.

Jesus is the most wonderful friend a person can ever have. A man who gave his life for me. What greater love is there than this?

Why did I ever doubt his love for me?

I go into the unknown over and over again knowing he is right there with me.

In so many ways I am a failure, but in Christ I am always a success — forgiven, loved and redeemed — that's the message …

I'm strolling down the path enjoying the peace and stillness of my heart.

This is only a porthole in the window of my soul.

3

I Am A New Creation

The familiar sound of the wheels under the bed as it rolled down the corridors of the Ulster Hospital — I was on my way to theatre.

'I'm going down here for a wee doze,' I said to the nurse who travelled with me on my journey.

I was crying my heart out, but as usual cracking jokes to put on a brave face. It was my fourth operation to remove yet more cancer from my mouth. There was barely a piece of flesh that hadn't been touched. I had been a smoker because I had so many problems in my life, one being schizophrenia. Thankfully I don't smoke anymore, but to be a regular on ward 4C is not something I ever thought would happen to me.

'God will never give me cancer,' I used to say. He knows I couldn't cope with it. Never underestimate the power and wisdom of God. I have learnt to trust and accept his decision on everything.

I was assigned a head and neck nurse to look after me. Her beauty was not only on the outside but deep within. She was such an amazing and gifted person. Her voice and general demeanour were extremely empathetic and compassionate. She understood difficult situations but always remained calm and very professional.

My consultant has been with me throughout my three-year journey. He has been a witness to all my moods. I will always be eternally grateful to him. He has given me back my life. What greater thing can any human being do?

My family and my friends have seen me laugh, and cry, in anger and in prayer. They have all been with me hand in hand on my journey. Including my dear friend Raymond, who was there for me one night when I was suicidal. I will never forget his words of comfort and reassurance.

Sarah, the blind girl I work for has strengthened and supported me throughout the last two years that I have been employed by her. She is not only the person I work for, but a very special friend.

Sadly lost two friends to cancer during my journey — Gemma and Sheila, and two friends Beverley and Simon, also died from other illnesses. When I lost these people in such a short space of time, I often wondered if I would be next. I have had such a traumatic life. 'I haven't even lived yet, I'm certainly not ready to die,' I say to myself often.

But it's an ill wind that blows no good. I have gone from a size sixteen/eighteen to a size twelve. When this happened, I gave all my clothes away to charity and some to friends.

I used to wear my hair short; I have grown it long. My old boss used to say to me that when I was thirty, my hair was my crowning glory. He said because I was a smoker, I would be lucky to see sixty, and he also said cigarettes wouldn't keep me out of heaven. He said they would just get me there more quickly.

In a few weeks I'm going to be sixty. I'm not a bit ashamed to say I dress like a thirty-year-old with my baseball boots, mom jeans, bomber jackets, and usually a big bow in my hair.

I don't care because when I was thirty, I dressed like a sixty-year-old. I don't deliberately dress to try and look young. I simply wear the clothes I love. I have a whole new wardrobe of clothes thanks to the love and generosity of my parents. I love to wear belts because for thirty years I was unable to.

I am a different person now, much more confident and I am loving being alive.

I have a wonderful husband who has been exceptional. His patience with me has been nothing less than outstanding. I am so fortunate to have him.

I don't know what my prognosis is, nor do I wish to. I leave my mouth cancer to the expertise of my consultant.

God has been faithful to me, but he has taught me a few very important lessons along the way; a number have been difficult lessons.

God has given me a second chance; he can do that for anyone. He did it through cancer. He really does work in mysterious ways.

Now, as I walk through the corridors of the hospital, it is to review appointments. Hopefully my days of trolley wheels are in the past.

And despite the uncertainty of my life expectancy, I am a new person. The old one has disappeared — and I really am a new creation.

4

Letting Go And Breaking China

I am sixty years old. My parents are still alive at the ages of eighty-eight and ninety-four. I consider myself fortunate to still have both my parents at my age.

This is my story about reaching out for things buried in the remotest and most inaccessible place in my heart, and how I am learning to let go of those things.

During my sixty years I have lost grandparents, a few friends and I have lost people I loved.

I had a boyfriend for a year when I was seventeen and I found painfully difficult to let go of him. I think I was hurting over the loss of him.

I know that someday I have to let go of my parents, unless they outlive me. When I was young, I don't think I could have coped. Now, I think I could cope in a way I couldn't have when I was younger.

I have had cancer for three years.

Letting go of my own life is something I used to rarely think about. Now it is something I think about every day. 'We all want to hang onto life,' my friend said to me. She's quite right, we do.

However, there is a battle going on in my head. I don't want to die, at least, not yet.

I am also schizophrenic, diagnosed at a young age. My life has been a life of sadness. Only God knows what I have been through; there must be comfort in that. But when I read that my life was planned out, I feel a real sense of hurt, a pain in my heart unlike any physical pain and I have often asked God, why?

Then I heard a story about a girl called Meghan, who was trafficked when she was a toddler.

At the age of thirty, she became free. She said she didn't need to be rescued; she needed to be received.

She had one year of happiness before she sadly died. I have no doubt there was an amazing peace in letting go and also tears of joy as she met her Saviour.

I realised after listening to Meghan's story that there are Christians out there, who have even sadder lives than mine.

Letting go of life does not need to be an emotionally painful experience. As Christians we are received at the other end.

God must feel the indescribable pain that I often feel. How often does he have to let go of people who reject his son? It must be the most painful experience that God must go through to have to look at a person he created and say to himself, it is time to let go.

I have not let go of my life yet, and God has blessed me with a fighting spirit; however, I have had to come through an extremely painful time of letting go a friend.

I did something. I made a mistake. I have apologised. Someone once said to me if you break a piece of your best friend's china, there is no need to keep repeatedly apologising to your friend. Your friend forgave you when it happened. So it should have been with the person who I thought was my friend. This is an illustration that we don't need to keep apologising to God.

Letting go of this friend is one of the most painful things I have ever had to do. The pain I felt reached the most remote and inaccessible place in my heart. I think a small part of me has died, and I don't think that void can be totally filled. But God has brought other people to me, blessed me with friends in abundance. It will hurt for a long time, but there is peace in being absorbed in things that give me pleasure. And God knows a sensitive heart and makes allowances for it.

When one door closes, another door opens, or as someone beautifully put it, when He closes a door, He opens a window.

It's about letting go of a chapter in your life and moving on to what God has in mind for you next. God knows each and every one of us intimately and knows how to heal our broken spirits and make us smile again. I find comfort in that; I hope you do too.

Don't worry if you break the china, it's when your heart breaks that God is waiting with his everlasting comforting arms.

Bull In A China Shop

As a Christian, I don't pay much attention to horoscopes. However, I do believe there is some truth in them and my star sign has certain characteristics which I believe relate specifically to me.

I was born on the third of May, so my star sign is Taurus, the bull. I am earthy, I love nature and natural colours, which I tend to keep using in my home, and in my wardrobe.

However, I am as stubborn as a bull, and I say I'm like a bull in a china shop. That doesn't mean I am tactless, on the contrary, I always consider people's feelings, but I have always been extremely outspoken and many people do not like it at all.

The Bible speaks about witnessing for The Lord. So, when I first got saved, I decided it was my duty to tell everyone, so every single person I met, was told that I had been saved. Several people, particularly non–Christians, looked embarrassed and didn't know how to answer, but on I went.

God handicapped me for many years with a serious mental illness, so I became subdued, and for many reasons I lacked confidence and was very low in self-esteem.

During my cancer journey, everything took a different turn. I lost all my excess weight, grew my hair long and started to take an interest in fashion; an interest which had been suppressed for years because of lack of money.

I have become an extremely confident person, but I hope I will never be described as *cocky* because that would be an insult.

After having cancer for two years, I left the City Hospital in December 2020. One day before I left, I looked at myself naked in a full-length mirror in my bathroom. It was after I had lost a lot of weight. I felt so happy, you could say I was tickled pink. Gone was the huge tummy. I will never have the perfect body, but it was an amazing moment.

The following year was a rollercoaster for me. I made friends and lost them. I behaved as though I was a bull in a china shop, and was extremely outspoken. After years of being put down, I decided there would be no more of that.

On reflection, I think being faced with a life-threatening illness made me reckless in many ways. It was as if I was saying, *I don't care, I'm going to die anyway; I will do and say whatever I like.*

But God only allowed this to go on for a while, because he is gracious, and then he said to me, *I'm going to teach you something, Alison.* Since then, many people have blocked me and abandoned me.

I still have many excellent friends, a supportive family and an amazingly patient husband.

I'm no longer a bull in a china shop, but in character, I'm as strong as a bull, make no mistake about that.

Thanks to God and my beautiful friend and saviour, the Lord Jesus Christ.

Schizophrenia
– The Unheard Voice

I was diagnosed with Schizophrenia in 1989. The events leading up to my diagnosis are no longer of any importance. They were unique, but we who suffer from this illness are all unique in our own special way.

The same as Kerry, with her mental illness, we are forgotten people. But we too have feelings, and hurts that run deep — we have not had it easy. I want to speak on behalf of all schizophrenics, because we are the unheard voice. I have schizophrenia.

When people hear you have been diagnosed with schizophrenia, they like to believe they have an understanding of your condition. However, it's complicated, and many people walk away. When you say something out of the ordinary, they are either going to laugh, gossip about you, block you on their phones, or else insult you badly, thereby wounding a person who has already been through the wars.

When I was first diagnosed with the illness, I lost every single friend I had. I was the gossip of the village where I lived. I witnessed people who claimed they were still my friends rolling their eyes when they saw me arrive at their door. Church people said they understood, but they never gave out their phone numbers, or invited me to their home for a cup of coffee. When Christ lived on this earth, he drank with tax collectors and harlots. He did not discriminate against anyone.

If Christ sat with me and I said something out of the ordinary, I believe he would have taken my hand and said, 'And Alison, how are you feeling when you say that?' He would say, 'Come dine with me and you can tell me all about it.'

I have since abandoned all the village people I used to like thirty years ago. One friend has remained — Christine. She is my best friend; she is true and loyal. Last year, during my cancer journey, every time I was waiting for an update on my diagnosis, unfortunately my coping mechanism was always to have a row with someone. I picked on anyone, but usually my nearest and dearest.

I felt as if I hated God, but I'm not allowed to, so I had to divert my anger and I knew the only people who would forgive me would be the people closest to me. So, I wrote nasty text messages to my friend Christine, who thankfully forgave me. It was all part of my mental state. Not only was I trying to cope with schizophrenia, but cancer had been thrown in too. Of course, I don't hate God. In fact, if Pastor

Steven Furtick, is right about what he tells us in his sermons, that the more you come up against the devil, it usually means you are doing something that is annoying him. If we live wishy-washy lives, the devil will leave us alone, because we are no threat to him. I worked for an elderly gentleman once called Neville. I addressed him as Mr, but his surname will remain confidential.

He was kind to me; I cleaned his house after his wife died. 'Come and sit down and tell me all your troubles,' he shouted at me every day when I was cleaning his kitchen. It was such an act of Christ. Then he died of cancer, but not before I told him he needed to be saved. Hopefully someday I will see him in Heaven. He did not discriminate, in fact, he reached out a loving hand. God bless Mr Neville.

We moved house twenty years ago and we live in a different town. I have made new, better friends. I never discriminate. A number of my friends are from different faiths, some are blind, others are mentally ill, some have cancer, some are just rejects of today's society. I love all my friends; they are unique and special in their own way. To all the schizophrenics out there, I'm writing this book, and if I ever earn enough money through my writing, I will support mental illness and cancer awareness. Cancer is not the worst thing that happened to me — that was schizophrenia.

7

A Guilty Conscience

Grace and I were friends as three year old's, well I was three, she was four. We lived at opposite ends of our street but found each other at a very early age and had a unique bond right from the start. We did everything together from dolls to tree huts.

One Christmas we sat in Grace's bedroom, we had probably been given fifty pence or a pound to buy Christmas presents, and we were working out what everyone would be receiving. A comb for Granny, a biro pen for Daddy etc.

We headed to the Supermac to do our Christmas shopping. On the way home we chatted with excitement about what wonderful presents we had bought. Eventually, we reached Grace's home and went straight to her bedroom to study our purchases.

After a short while Grace looked puzzled. 'I don't think I was charged for everything,' she said. 'I wasn't charged for the Old Spice talc.' We looked at each other, two little girls thinking the same thing. I honestly don't remember who spoke, but one of us said, 'We could do this again, obviously no one even noticed.' We were tempted to go back and steal next time.

A week passed and on Friday night we set off. We reached the Supermac and in we went. I don't know what Grace stole, but I had my eye on a packet of coloured pencils. I hovered around looking and watching. At last my chance came, and into my pocket they went. I looked around — nobody had seen.

Shortly after, we left the supermarket and started our journey home. It was a fifteen-minute walk. After walking for about five minutes, I had an overwhelming feeling of guilt. All that my mummy and daddy had taught me came flooding back. I told Grace I had to go back. She went on home. So, back I went to the counter of the Supermac, and when I was satisfied that no one was looking, I replaced the pencils. It was such a feeling of relief. I had learnt a very important lesson, and no harm had been done, or so I thought.

I journeyed home as a happy little girl. That night I felt I had to tell my mummy because I told her everything. I was shocked at her response. She was angry and unforgiving. Thankfully, eventually she made peace with me, but the incident had a negative effect on me and my mum who has always loved me without a shadow of a doubt. Perhaps she had reasons for her reaction. Did she did not realise that me, a young sensitive child would grow up and have many mental problems? Of course, I don't have any bitterness about the event or about my mum. I love her dearly. My life was mapped out a long time ago. It was meant to happen for a reason and we all know God always brings good from the most trialing of circumstances. It says so in the Bible and I believe it.

I'm sixty now and Mum and I couldn't be closer. I am a Christian, so forgiving my mum is not difficult. God allowed it to happen, so I could tell my story today. If a mum is reading this, be gentle on your child. It's so important. God is very gentle on us.

8

Home From Home

There is something extremely comforting about lying snuggled up under the blankets in a caravan listening to the patter of rain on the roof, and the intermittent sound of the lighthouse foghorn.

I'm at my favourite place in the whole world, Cranfield. Today is my sixtieth birthday. The caravan is luxurious in comparison to the caravans we had when I was a teenager in exactly the same place, but Cranfield Bay, a beach with two headlands, still looks exactly the same, fifty years later.

The old place conjures up memories of first kisses, romances, fun and games, and people who have disappeared out of my life forever. I often wonder how their lives turned out.

They are different people now, which leaves a sadness, a kind of ache in my heart, a longing to meet up with those people who played a huge part in my youth.

People and places make life; that's what I think.

I have new people in my life now, people in the hometown where I live, which again is different to the place where I was brought up.

I've been living with cancer for the past three years. We bought the caravan when I became ill, and what a beautiful and unselfish thing my husband did. He knew how much it meant to me.

We often either drive or walk to the castle that is about a mile from the caravan site. Who used to live there? That's another story about someone else's life. The remains of the castle are still standing and you can climb up high and look out to Carlingford Lough that stretches a long way in the distance.

We climbed the castle as children, and we climbed the castle as teenagers.

Now that I'm sixty I have no desire to climb those steps, but I love that old castle.

We've owned this caravan for three years but barely know anyone because of Covid and also the past three summers have been taken up with surgery, either having, or waiting for or recovering from it.

This year I am hoping to enjoy Cranfield.

Sometimes, I just love to be in the caravan. There is a muffled sound of voices as people walk past. I have my music which

I love to listen to and I'm surrounded by photos of children and grandchildren.

Today is my birthday. Because of my mouth cancer, I can no longer eat properly, so we won't be celebrating by going out for a meal.

No, it's shopping today, not grocery shopping. It's retail therapy, all the lovely things that I probably don't need. But that will only take a couple of hours.

I plan a lovely walk along the beach. I can still hear the music playing at the beach disco when I was ten, and remember paddling home, feet at the edge of the water singing along to the music of the seventies and being met by our parents who were worried because we were out so late.

It was such a safe environment in those days. It was an idyllic place.

I hope I keep my caravan for the rest of my life. Sadly, my children don't have the same feelings about Cranfield.

It is special to me. It's my favourite place on earth. I have never travelled in my life. I didn't desire or need to. I have all I need here at Cranfield.

9

Kerry

It was late one Wednesday afternoon at the end of August, I was so keen to get ready for the pop-up shop, which I would be running for a week at the beginning of October. I was on Facebook every night looking for bargains to sell with my upcycling. On Tuesday night, I texted a girl regarding three metres of material that she was selling. It turned out to be the end of a roll. Raspberry pink and green, a beautiful combination.

So on Wednesday, I stopped at our local garage to withdraw some money. I also had an ottoman to pick up in East Belfast … I knew my timing was bad; I was just about to hit rush-hour traffic.

I parked at the garage near the side wall of the shop. I noticed a young girl sitting on the pavement slouched in a position that seemed to say, I'm here for a while, but I hope I get a lift home.

She was dressed in jeans. She was quite petite with a black baseball cap, and long-dark hair, her curly lips were beautifully painted in raspberry pink.

Under her cap, she looked as if she was talking to herself. I stood by the car. She didn't notice me watching her. I thought she looked a bit vulnerable and lost ...

I marched over to the cashpoint, but all the way, I felt God saying to me, never mind your material, get that wee girl sorted. I came back to my car.

'Are you okay?' I asked her.

'Yes,' she said as she looked up.

'Have you got a lift home?' I said.

'Yes, well no, actually, I live on the Woodstock Road,' she replied as she lifted her head.

I know some people will think I was crazy, but I spoke to God immediately and said, *I'm taking this girl home, protect me Lord.*

'I'll take you home, jump in; but we have an errand to do on the way,' I said to her. She stood up immediately and we both got into the car. I explained I was picking up material at Carryduff, but I would be heading to East Belfast afterwards.

Her name was Kerry. I didn't ask why she was in Comber. I was interested in her, but I'm neither nosey nor judgmental. I knew she was either high on drugs or afflicted by the side effects of medication. She told me she was thirty-two years old, unmarried, but she had a boyfriend. She had been abandoned by her mother at a very young age, but had contact with her father. She had no home, was mentally ill and unable to work, but was looked after by Social Services. She had no children. She actually looked about twenty-two.

Her mobile phone seemed to be bigger than the standard one. She chatted and played music.

'I want to give you a song,' she said.

'Oh lovely, play it to me,' I replied. She played Sun Kil Moon and their song *Ålesund*. It was a lovely relaxing piece of music.

As our journey progressed I told her a bit about me, how I had become a Christian through the strangest of circumstances, what had set the wheels in motion to me getting saved. I told her God loved her and not to be put off Christianity by the stereotype women in crimplene dresses with fancy hats who go to church every Sunday, because a lot of them don't live in the real world. However, I happen to know that these women have their stories too.

Eventually, we reached the Cregagh Road. She asked me to give her a song, so I posted one on Facebook every night. The first one I chose was *Footprints in the Sand* by Leona Lewis. She played it for a while but seemed to get bored. Eventually we reached the Woodstock Road.

'Oh,' she said. 'Just let me out here.' She gathered her few things, got out and disappeared. I have no idea where she lived or her surname.

Kerry is one of the forgotten people, through no fault of her own, but she is a person with feelings — like you and me. And she has gifts like you and me that need to be brought out.

I'm glad I took her home; I wouldn't have missed that journey for the world. Hopefully, someday in eternity, Jesus will call over me and say, 'Here is a friend of yours Alison, its Kerry.'

I told my daughter, Rachael, the story. She gave me a song to put up on Facebook that night and I put up, To Kerry and the song, *Does Anybody Hear Her* by Casting Crowns. It's a song about people such as Kerry — they are all over the world. You might meet a Kerry yourself one day. Don't walk past. Reach out the hand that Jesus reached out to you.

10

Life Can Be Cruel

The bell rang at 8.50 a.m. The whole school made their way to assembly. It was September, my first day in an all-girls grammar school.

I had left primary school in June and with me came one friend. We stuck together as kids do and soon after the year began another girl joined us.

I have often pondered during many years of my life about the reason for the fall out. But still, to this day I can't remember. At some point both of these girls suddenly abandoned me.

I was lucky being a person who made friends easily, but unfortunately on this occasion, I did not choose wisely. I got myself into the company of girls who were not workers. They were just passing their time. There was one I was particularly close to.

After religious education one day I turned to her and said, 'Do you think I'm a Christian?' Her reaction is something I will never forget. She laughed, mocked me and imitated my voice.

It's funny how I can't remember what I did last night, but the memory of that is rooted deeply in my mind. School was very difficult and although I am an intelligent person, I did not do well. I came away from school a shy, awkward person, greatly lacking in confidence, even though I was blossoming into a pretty girl.

I had my first boyfriend when I was sixteen. The break-up was difficult and one night when I went out for a walk alone to clear my head, I was attacked by a man and dragged over a wall and sexually assaulted. He was never caught.

I met my husband at the age of nineteen when I was a model. He has many special qualities. He is humble, kind, loyal, affectionate and very caring. He was so proud of me.

At a fashion show one night in one of the top hotels in Belfast, he must have nudged everyone around him and pointed to the catwalk. 'That's my fiancée,' he said.

We were married in 1983, but hit hard times and five years and two children later, I went to a solicitor for a divorce.

Before I knew what was happening, I was in the middle of an affair with this solicitor. The affair humbled me, and one night in tears, thankfully I turned to God for help.

Sadly, the whole episode had already taken its toll. I was seriously mentally ill and after a ten-week stay in a psychiatric unit, my husband was told I was schizophrenic. I was twenty-seven years old.

Many difficult years lay ahead. With the medication I put on a lot of weight, especially round my tummy. 'When is your baby due?' I was asked constantly.

My confidence took another blow.

I was treated badly by many people, put down and as soon as people heard my diagnosis, I was not listened to or treated with any respect. Even my family were guilty. I felt so hurt and so alone.

I have one lovely friend who has stood by me all these years through it all. My Christian friend Christine is such a special person.

After I turned forty, we moved house and life started to improve. I had a few pleasant years.

Working for a cancer charity as a fundraiser helped my confidence, but I still wasn't able to stand up for myself. My problem was deep rooted.

I was a heavy smoker and the addiction had really got hold of me; however, I did stop smoking in 2014, but five years later, I received another blow — mouth cancer.

In the town where I lived, at this stage in my life, I had made a lot of friends.

I have had four operations on my mouth and I have also had chemotherapy and radiotherapy.

During my stay in the City Hospital, I found it strange to be told that I was a model patient by my senior consultant. He said I was easy to get on with, very co-operative, polite to everyone and appreciated all that was being done for me.

My friends were all praying for me and telling me how proud they were of me; how I handled my illness so well and with great courage.

Five of them sewed and knitted beautiful gifts for me. I was overwhelmed at the love I felt. Something amazing was happening.

My confidence was beginning to grow. I was moving away from being a shy, awkward person who had nothing to say and no self-esteem.

Suddenly, I was able to stand up for myself. I was tired of being treated badly. Suddenly I found my voice and now I use it when I need to.

People no longer walk over me. I like to think I give everyone a fair chance. But nobody will ever put me down again.

Cancer is by no means the worst thing that has ever happened to me. I might not be able to speak as I once did, but in many ways, I much prefer my new voice. Its kind, loving, sensitive, appreciative and I am so pleased to say assertive.

This is the beauty of our God, the greatest counsellor of all. Yes, life can be cruel but our God is greater.

11

A Moment Of Madness

It was the beginning of December, Paddy and I strolled in the park; it was 11 p.m. I can't even remember where we were coming from.

Paddy and I were best friends, next-door neighbours; we met in our teens when we were seventeen and knew each other well.

A car drew up at the end of my driveway. The window rolled down.

'Fancy a spin?' said a guy in the passenger seat.

I looked more closely and saw my ex-boyfriend in the back of the car. We had split up the previous Easter. I wasn't really over him.

I looked at Paddy. 'What do you think?' I said.

She looked warily at me. 'Not me,' she replied.

'Well, I'm going,' I said. A moment of madness. It was because only eight months previously I had been out walking one night, close to home, when a man dragged me over a wall, stripped me and sexually assaulted me.

I went into my house and told my mum I was having supper with Paddy, and I might be late. Off I went.

Can't remember much about the chat on the way to Newtownards. They took me to a pub. We had to climb steps.

One of the guys I knew vaguely through my ex-boyfriend. He kept buying me drinks. I was quite drunk when we left the pub.

We drove, and I chatted away and I sang songs.

Suddenly we stopped, they had noticed an abandoned car. They got out and apparently struggled without success to remove the stereo system from the car. We drove on. I was neither frightened nor nervous. I have no idea why?

At Kirkliston racing track we stopped again. All four got out.

My ex-boyfriend got into the seat beside me. Well, there was no mistaking what he wanted, but I told him no and he did not try to force me. He got out, another one got in. Repeat. The answer was quite definitely NO.

We drove further down the road with me singing rude songs that I can no longer remember. It was then about two a.m.

As we approached East Belfast, the one who had been buying me drinks whispered in my ear. 'I'll meet you in the Rosetta Bar tomorrow night at 6 p.m.' I was quite taken aback. I looked closely at him. He was a handsome guy. 'Okay,' I said and nodded.

The driver dropped them all off and told me to sit in the front seat ... he took me to my door. 'I think you're a great person, great craic, I would love to take you out sometime,' he said before I got out. I was taken aback again. 'But you have a girlfriend,' I replied. I stepped out of the car and never saw him again.

I only dated the other guy for a month.

It was a moment of madness. I didn't tell my mum until years after I got married. It was probably one of the silliest and the most daring things I have ever done.

Regardless, it still makes me smile.

At a time in my life when I was speedily approaching mental illness, God gave me a night of fun, and all the while, he was watching over me, making sure I came to no harm.

Where are those people now? What did they do with their lives? I'll never know, at least, not in this world.

Poems

NOT READY TO DIE

On a cold November day, to the dentist I did go

A tiny flap of skin was what I had to show

Johnny looked into my mouth to
see this tiny flap

We'll do a wee biopsy and see what comes of that

Inconclusive is what came back

The hospital wanted to see

I had no idea at that point the
journey in front of me

The consultant took a better look with his
well-trained eye

It doesn't look like very much

We'll see you again in a while

Three or four times later, another
flap would show

Soon it became apparent that the cancer
had begun to grow

Four operations later and three
years down the line

Every day I say to myself, is this now my time?

But every time a lump appears, or something's
not quite right

The Lord is whispering to me, please don't
give up the fight

For He has reminded me often, how
precious I am to Him

Still on earth I am right now, the place
he wants me to be

There is still work to be done and
willing and able am I

I am not ready to leave this world yet, no, I am
not ready to die

There are things I want to do; things I
want to achieve

Things I have not yet experienced

I am nowhere near ready to leave

So I leave my life with the Lord, and any
cancer, I leave with him too

The Lord will always do the right thing, I leave
it all with him, I really do

Praise our Lord God, Praise the Lord Jesus too

However I am tested,
I depend ultimately on you.

TO A SPECIAL FRIEND

As Helena Steiner Rice once told

A story about the windows of gold

I have my own version which now I will share

And no longer this burden do I have to bear

For happy am I, I have been set free

From chains that for a long time,
  were holding me

I often felt lonely, burdened and sad

Complaining of things that I never had

When all of a sudden with cancer I fell

And this is now the story I tell

The Lord is my shepherd, I shall not want

How true are these words to the finest point

Searching was I for that window of gold

This is the story of how God's grace can unfold

Searching was I, foolish in my way

When all I needed to do was pray

Friends I have many, all special to me

But one stands out as the speciality

And no, a lover he will never be

He's a million times more special to me

Dripping from his tongue are
words I love to hear

His choices, his values, his kind
and listening ear

A friend true and kind, loyal and faithful is he

All the qualities I admire which are
very special to me

The void is completely filled and
happy is my soul

No longer do I complain, I am now
completely whole

I no longer need to look at the
far window of gold

I'll have everything I'll ever need or
want with my Lord

He has given me a husband so
gentle and so dear

Children and grandchildren
who draw very near

Parents who have loved me, and that
love has no end

Countless people surround me and count me
as their friend

The window of gold is not a distant thing

Because I have lived my life trusting in the King

That special person is here, and I
did not even see

When I first met him, how special
he would be to me

He has a lovely wife, and blessed is she

But his friendship is what is important to me

I'm happy to be tenth or twentieth down the line

I'm here as his friend, whenever he has the time

Happy am I, my soul is set free

The Lord God has always been very good to me

The window of gold is not a faraway land

This little piece of gold is right here at my hand

For prayers answered Lord, I praise
and worship too

"Cast your burden on the Lord, for he
careth for you."

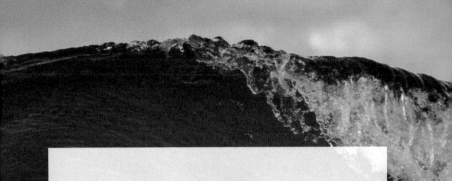

TO ALLY

What a courageous lady you are

*Your acceptance of your condition
inspirational by far*

*Your prayers will be answered in a
most caring way*

*I'm sure the Good Lord will gently
guide you day by day*

Written by Alf Fell

MUM AND ME

*The first time we bonded was when I was
lovingly soothed within your womb as I listened
to the thud of a marvellous beat*

*And then I was born, held and spoken to by you,
and oh what a sound, your voice so sweet*

*I remember the days when you walked me
to and collected me from school, I would
hug you so tight …*

*After all the days/years of being bullied I knew
as soon as you held me in your arms everything
would be alright*

So, the years went by and I grew

*You comforted me when my heart had been
broken by boys*

*And you reassured me that someone very special
would come later down the line*

*When I was nineteen we sat and we prayed that
within three years I would meet my husband*

*He came into our lives a year before that
deadline had passed … so just in time*

*Then came your precious grandsons and our
hearts were overcome with love*

The way they look at you Mum, bonds so
beautiful to see

It is clear as a family we were very
much meant to be

So, then you and me went through
something unexpected

Chronic illnesses in both of us had
sadly been detected

But through pain and various surgeries we have
held each other up

Many prayers and much love, we
have never given up

Each day comes with its own challenges,
each day we see each other's strength, courage
and resilience

I wish we didn't have to go through what we do

But if I had to go through it with anyone who I
knew could cope, it would be you

I know you love butterflies Mum

So I will tell you a little secret

Our bodies are like a caterpillar's cocoon ...
each day they become a little more brittle

But even when the last piece of our
cocoon is broken

And we leave this life

We will come forth a body new, a butterfly so
beautiful, wings so strong

As the journey is made towards
our eternal home.

After another cancer diagnosis this week Mum

We hope and pray your cocoon continues to stay
strong for many years

But someday when we have to part, it
won't be forever

It will just be, I'll see you again someday.

Yes, there may be tears, but boy will there be a
celebration of this woman my mother who has
always been so strong, as this beautifully created
butterfly spreads her new wings and arrives at
her forever heavenly home.

Love you always Mum, your
daughter Rachael xo

MY SPECIAL FRIEND

My special friend walks past my heart

And smiles, but drops a kiss on my soul

My special friend is someone I text in the middle of the night

And get a reply a few minutes later

My special friend is never too busy to talk

My special friend arrives in a cardigan she hasn't got around to sewing buttons on

And I see nothing but beauty

My special friend does not gossip about other people

My special friend makes me laugh

My special friend is on my side

My special friend knows the longings of my heart and keeps it to herself

My special friend knows I'm ill and ignores the dust in my house

My special friend knows I love her

My special friend never takes advantage of me

My special friend knows I am vulnerable

My special friend knows I have different moods

My special friend will be at my funeral

I hope all my special friends will join me in heaven.

GRIEF

When your train has stopped at the darkest,
most deserted place on earth and you are alone

When you remove your glasses for the hundredth
time to wipe the tears from your eyes and you
realise it's better to leave them off for today

When you can't even think of a time
when you were happy

When an alcoholic drink is your best friend and
also your worst enemy

When you realise you've been staring at the same
ornament for an hour

When life going on around you is as far removed
from you as the earth is to the sun

When you don't actually want to die, but being
alive is just too painful

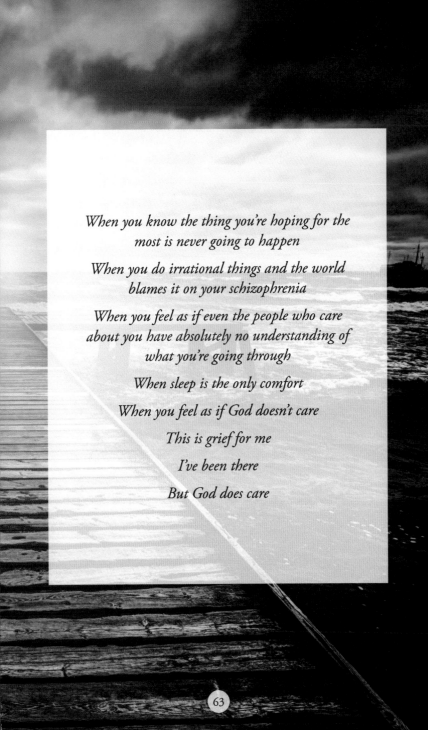

When you know the thing you're hoping for the
most is never going to happen

When you do irrational things and the world
blames it on your schizophrenia

When you feel as if even the people who care
about you have absolutely no understanding of
what you're going through

When sleep is the only comfort

When you feel as if God doesn't care

This is grief for me

I've been there

But God does care

NEVER BY GOD

I have been hurt by loved ones

But never by God

I have been insulted

But never by God

I have been put down

But never by God

I have had my heart broken

But never by God

I have been disappointed

But never by God

I have been abandoned

But never by God

I have been hated

I have only ever been loved by God.

FOUR STRONG WOMEN

Tribute to my mum, two sisters
and my daughter
They are all so different
Walking different paths
The four closest women to me
They all know me well
They know all my faults
I know all theirs too
But we are all walking in the same direction
The four of them holding me up
The weak one
None of them are mentally ill or have cancer
But they all have a deep understanding
Of my complex needs
We have friendship
We laugh together
They are sad with me
They all love me
And I love all of them
None of them have ever let me down
They are there
They will never leave me or forsake me.

WE THREE SISTERS

Here we three are at the caravan again

The sunshine and soft breeze
have turned to rain

Another summer is saying goodbye

Slowly disappearing with a heave and a sigh

The campsite is empty, they will soon all be gone

Back to school and work, the season is done

The beach is empty, only a few to be seen

The lifeguards are idle, they who
once were so keen

The shop is almost bare, they all stand and wait

The office is quiet, all waiting for the date

But we three are here to say our farewell

To sister Hilary, whose company has been swell

Home from Australia, three months have flown

Good times we've had, seeds have been sewn

Fifty years on from the first time we were here

So much has happened over those years

But we three are solid, withstanding life's storm

The bond that we have can never be torn

This caravan holds stories and
laughter and tears

Which will withstand the weather in
the twilight years

We will grow old together, even though far apart

Bonded together by the veins of our heart

The season is over, autumn is near

We three sisters hold each other so dear.

I AM THE GEEK

*The wolf in sheep's clothing with
words oh so sweet*

Sometimes makes me forget that I am the geek

Eccentric and different, a non-mainstream lass

*A pretty little face, charming, and with
a touch of class*

*But oh, I have a marriage, and
jealous are my friends*

*A man who would give his life for me, a love
that has no end*

*Did Christ not do that too? I ask
myself in total shock*

Was Billy sent by an angel?

It wasn't just good luck

*No, God had a special plan, and
thankfully I see it now*

No longer am I in the dark

My marriage is as special as Thou

*I admire Dr H and Chris, so
wonderful they are to me*

They let me scream and fight and kick

Until the truth I eventually see

But abandon me, they do not, and more
than thankful am I

I am the Geek, after all, and their
patience I do try

But God is always in control and
understanding of me is he

My loving nature melts his heart, and only
through Christ I see

How blessed I am, to have a father so good

And a husband like Billy to put
up with my moods

Friends in abundance, especially
Christine and Chris

Strangely they have been given the same name,
that certainly wasn't a mistake

So for all my kicks and screams, I am thankful
for true friends

I am the non-stream charming lass, whose
appreciation never ends

TO MY HUSBAND (BILLY)

On one August we met at a dance

The beginning of a beautiful romance

His dark sultry eyes flashed across the floor

My baby blue ones glanced back to
say I wanted more

The end of the summer in a seaside town

Of beautiful Newcastle, in County Down

We had walks in the country

Made love in the car

I knew at the very beginning

He was a special person by far

He was a farm labourer by trade

Not a very well paid job

Big, strong, well-tanned hands

Working class, but not a yob

No, a kind, caring, loving, gentle man was he

Raised in a big family by his mother alone

A grafter he was known as far and wide

The hardest working man with a heart of corn

And married we were in 1983

Two years later, wee ones on my knee

Hit hard times and grew far apart

Only the beginning of the breaking of my heart

The rest is history, my friends all know the score

A lot of it is private, and not for me to share

But God lifted me out of the miry clay

Washed me in the blood, and
gave me a new day

So now I am a Christian and proud
to say the name

Schizophrenia and cancer have met
me along the way

And many other problems, no two the same

But God has never let me down, I
really need to say

We're in our sixties now with our
marriage thru the mill

Billy has been strong and steadfast in every way

A tower of strength with the patience of a saint

I thank my Heavenly Father for him
every single day.

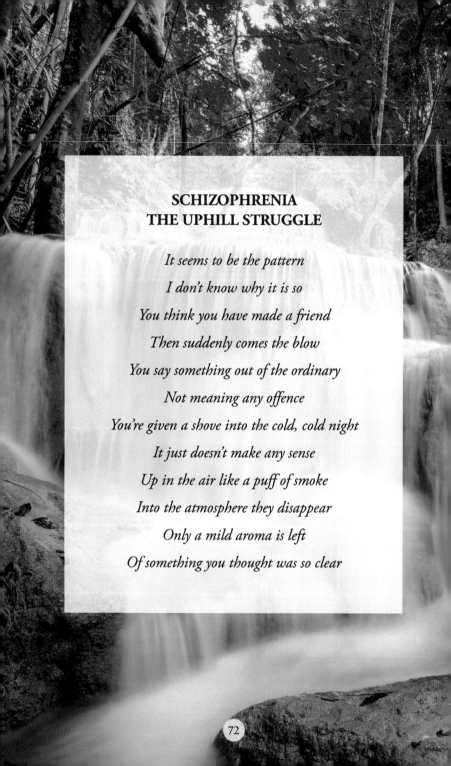

SCHIZOPHRENIA
THE UPHILL STRUGGLE

It seems to be the pattern

I don't know why it is so

You think you have made a friend

Then suddenly comes the blow

You say something out of the ordinary

Not meaning any offence

You're given a shove into the cold, cold night

It just doesn't make any sense

Up in the air like a puff of smoke

Into the atmosphere they disappear

Only a mild aroma is left

Of something you thought was so clear

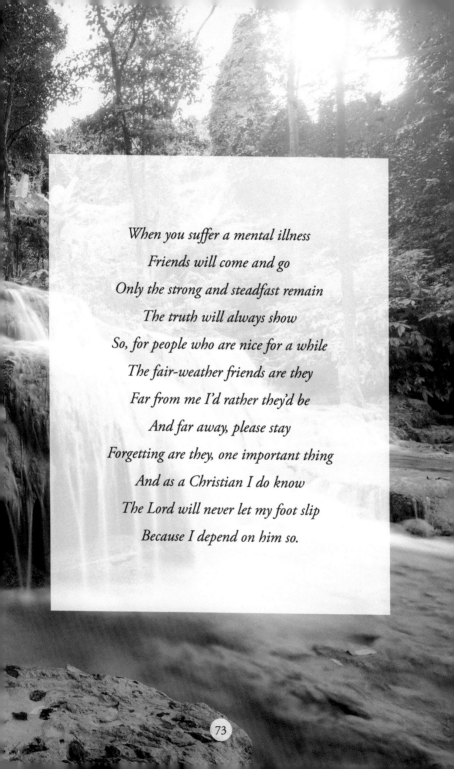

When you suffer a mental illness
Friends will come and go
Only the strong and steadfast remain
The truth will always show
So, for people who are nice for a while
The fair-weather friends are they
Far from me I'd rather they'd be
And far away, please stay
Forgetting are they, one important thing
And as a Christian I do know
The Lord will never let my foot slip
Because I depend on him so.

The End.

CONTACT THE AUTHOR
author.alison.murphy@gmail.com

INSPIRED TO WRITE A BOOK?

Contact

Maurice Wylie Media

Inspirational & Christian Book Publisher

Based in Northern Ireland and distributing
around the world.

www.MauriceWylieMedia.com